Using Arthritis Against Itself

Finding a pain-free life
from inside a life in pain

BRYDON DAVIDSON

First published 2022 by Brydon Davidson

Produced by Indie Experts P/L, Australasia
indieexperts.com.au

Cover design by Daniela Catucci @ Catucci Design
Edited by Anne-Marie Tripp
Internal design by Indie Experts
Typeset in 10/17 pt Metropolis by Post Pre-press Group, Brisbane

ISBN 978-0-473-62101-8 (paperback)
ISBN 978-0-473-62103-2 (hardcover)
ISBN 978-0-473-62105-6 (epub)
ISBN 978-0-473-62106-3 (kindle)

Dedicated to the strength of all those who live with an autoimmune disease. No one will ever know nor understand the yoke of pain you joust with every minute of every day of every year . . . on top of just trying to live your lives . . . all the while hoping science and medicine find the answer.

Respect.

Contents

How it all began

In mid-2003, my life changed significantly.

I was living in Port Moresby, Papua New Guinea, and working as a manager in Deloitte (a 'Big Four' accounting firm).

At the time, I was a fit, strong, and active 35-year-old male enjoying life. When I wasn't working, I was having fun travelling the world and doing a lot of physical activities, including snowboarding, dancing in nightclubs (techno is my thing), rollerblading, some rock climbing, kayaking, hiking, lifting weights, swimming, cycling, and coaching as well as playing touch rugby when in season.

Standing 1.88 metres tall, weighing 85 kilograms, and with somewhere between 5 and 10% body fat, my body and I had what I thought was a healthy relationship. I looked after it by feeding it good food, exercising and resting it, just as I'd done since I was a teenager. And in return, my body gave me the freedom to do pretty much anything I wanted without too much discomfort – and, bonus, it wasn't unattractive to the opposite sex.

But in mid-2003, everything changed and my body stopped responding to exercise as it had in the past. At the time, I was coaching and training our firm's touch rugby team, hoping to win the annual inter-firm touch footy tournament again for the fourth year in a row.

For those of you who haven't been to Papua New Guinea, you need to know that it's always hot and depending on the season it's either very dry or very wet. The tournament was always held in the dry season, so at the time of, and leading up to the tournament event, the ground was usually dry and very hard. That's tough on a big body.

I normally got shin splints from running on hard ground, so I always prepared to reduce the damage by buying good footwear and using some recovery 'tricks' after training to help my bones and joints heal quicker. But that year, the tricks didn't work. Where normally I would be able to start the next training session with good shins, I was training with sore shins that hadn't recovered from the last training.

My ribs also hurt a lot during and after training. I always pushed myself, but I couldn't understand why my chest hurt so much just from running and nothing else – it wasn't like I was being tackled.

These discomforts grew and grew, and by the time of the final I was on anti-inflammatories just to get through the competition – something I'd never had to do before. We ended up winning, which was good, but it wasn't fun doing it in pain.

With the tournament over, I turned my attention to giving my body a good chance to recover. I was able to successfully make my shin splints go away. But no matter what I did, I couldn't do the same for my chest pains.

It was a weird pain. It's hard to explain what it was like, but the best I can do is tell you it felt like my ribs were being crushed in a vice and at the same time I felt like I was being ripped apart. Like I said, it was weird!

On top of that, as I slowly tried to return to the other physical exercises I used to do, small injuries that previously would have gone away in a few weeks never seemed to resolve.

I was now battling pain and inflammation more often than not. The normal strategies I used to recover from injuries or muscle pain (ice packs, heat packs, traction, chiropractors, physio) didn't seem to be working at all.

Using Arthritis Against Itself

After months of being unable to solve my pain problem myself, I started seeing doctors – first in Papua New Guinea and then offshore in Australia. I spent over a year seeing various doctors, trying to work out what the hell was going on with my body. After many false diagnoses (one doctor thought I might have pleurisy, an inflammation of the tissue around the lungs), the conclusion was that I was dealing with arthritis.

Initially I rejected the idea that it could be arthritis. I mean, seriously? Arthritis is an old person's disease, right? I was a 35-year-old who was fit and active, ate well, exercised regularly, and looked after myself – basically doing everything you're supposed to do to be and stay healthy. It couldn't be arthritis. The doctors had to be wrong.

The thing is, it didn't really matter if the doctors were right or wrong. All that mattered was that I was living with pain every day. By then, I had stopped almost all physical exercise because my joints, muscles and tendons weren't working anywhere near what they used to. I was in constant pain almost everywhere in my body, with my ribs and my neck being the worst (I was having trouble turning my neck at all).

The sooner I accepted what the doctors were telling me, the sooner I could stop fighting against whatever diagnosis

I had been given, and instead focus on what I was going to do about my body being constantly in pain.

I recall it took me around six months to stop fighting, and accept what the doctors were telling me. And it was only then that I was able to change my focus from finding ways to prove the doctors wrong to instead finding out as much as I could about arthritis to better understand what it might be and, in theory, how I might beat it.

I continued to follow the doctors' referrals to help gather more information (and eliminate things that weren't relevant). This concluded with me seeing a rheumatologist who was pretty confident that I had a specific type of arthritis – ankylosing spondylitis.

His prognosis was that I would have to live with this for the rest of my life – with constant pain that at best could be reduced but never eliminated, with progressively stronger pain meds and the side effects that come with them. The only other option, depending on where my pain was coming from, was surgeries to fuse joints to stop the pain.

To say that I was angry about this would be an understatement. While I didn't have my future planned out, the idea of living any life constantly in pain and at the mercy of pain meds was pretty unappealing.

If I wanted a different future than the specialists and the doctors were describing to me, then it was up to me to find a way, because according to them, this was now my life. There was no cure.

And so began my journey of facing my arthritis head on (without any knowledge of whether I could beat it, or if it might go away), concluding in me beating my arthritis three years later in July 2006 . . . and it not since returning.

Ever since I beat my arthritis, I have been asked a number of times how I did it. This book is my answer to that question.

If you are going to do something you have never done, aim for something you cannot see, I believe it is super important to have some fundamental principles you can rely on to guide you. Think of them as your compass in a world where you have no map. Without them you will falter.

For me, the answer lay within the following five fundamental principles I chose to guide me:

1 Doctors and specialists don't know everything about all sicknesses and all human bodies. They just work with what they know and not what they don't know (presumably so they avoid giving people false hope). People have cured themselves of other ailments despite a specialist's best

prognosis. And while it is true they may be the exception, that does not mean we should ignore those minorities and their successes entirely. So if someone else was able to cure themselves of an ailment despite being told it couldn't happen, I could do the same with my arthritis.

2 I wasn't living in pain before I was 35, so if something happened to 'turn my arthritis on', then it must be able to be turned off, too. The fact that specialists don't really know what turns arthritis on in some people (and therefore don't know how to turn it back off) wasn't going to stop me trying to discover this for myself.

3 I had nothing to lose – at worst, the specialists would be correct and I would live in pain the rest of my life. And at best (if I could find my answer), I might actually cure myself of arthritis and be pain-free again. And even if I didn't achieve being pain-free, I might find ways to reduce the pain I had to endure enough to reduce my reliance on medication, or slow down my progression to stronger meds. Win-win!

4 Anything is possible as long as you want it enough. I really wanted to be pain-free again, and not live in pain the rest of my life, so I accepted

I would try anything and everything that could help me towards my goal – regardless of how uncomfortable, unpleasant, or weird it might be. There had to be no regrets. There couldn't be any doubt I tried something properly, just because I may not believe in it or because it was uncomfortable. It would have been tragic to try something half-assed and it not work . . . but it would have worked if I had tried it properly. I only had one condition – the potential cure couldn't be worse than the arthritis itself.

5 The body can cure itself but we have to let it – sometimes it's not what you do but what you stop doing that matters. Sometimes we're busy doing things that get in the way of things we want, and that applies to how we live, what we eat, and how we feed our bodies. Removing bad habits, wrong thinking patterns, bad food, and bad thoughts provides more energy and less blockages, allowing the body to heal itself.

With those five principles in mind, I started exploring myths, ideas, research, anecdotal evidence, stories – anything that might help me understand better what was going on in my body, and ultimately (hopefully) cure myself of this scourge of a disease. And with the research I gradually uncovered, I began to experiment on myself.

Disclaimer

If it isn't already clear, I'm no doctor – I have no education nor qualifications in the medical industry. I also do not know your medical history, nor do I know who you are as a person.

I wrote this book to share my experiences and to offer hope to those enduring 24/7 pain from arthritis or other auto-immune problems.

Because everyone is unique, it's impossible for me to know whether or not you will achieve the same outcome as me even if you follow my journey.

Therefore, I must make 100% sure you understand the following:

- This book you're reading now was created for informational purposes only and provides general information and discussion about arthritis and related subjects. Nothing shared in this book is to be taken as professional advice with regards to health or any other field.

- Everything contained in this book reflects my personal experiences, observations, opinions and methods used to find my way through arthritis.

- Seek medical advice from a licensed professional, physician or healthcare worker before making any changes to your lifestyle, diet or treatment program. While I may not have sought medical advice prior to trying some of the strategies I used to ultimately recover from my arthritis, I urge you to not do the same. I was lucky. In hindsight, I put myself at more risk by not discussing some of my strategies with my doctors and specialists beforehand.

- If you think you may have a medical emergency, call your doctor or your relevant emergency number immediately (111 in New Zealand).

With that out of the way, you can now learn the things I did that I believe contributed to me beating my arthritis . . . and hopefully find your own path along the way.

Where to start?

When I started my journey to finding my way through my arthritis, I had no map. I had no guide. And, if I listened to my doctors and specialists, I had no hope.

Facing the unknown and having to live with pain 24/7, I did the only thing I've ever done when I'm having a bad day, week or month. I just put one foot in front of the other and soldiered on. It's the only way I know how to make sure I am moving forward when times are tough.

I know from experience that things will always get better as long as I keep moving forward . . . regardless of how I feel. And if whatever I'm doing gets worse, I change course. And conversely, if things get better, I keep doing what I'm doing.

So I started with my diet because food and nutrition had been such a big part of my life as a fit and active person.

I strongly believe that you are what you eat, and food is medicine, so it seemed like the most logical place to start. While I played around with my diet, I also looked for ways to conserve my energy, and I also worked on educating my friends, family and workmates.

I was able to work on three things at once without any problems because:

- I have never been one to do anything half-assed. If I do anything, I give it my all regardless of what happens. My mind is way stronger than my body, which means I can push myself forward even when my body thinks it doesn't want to.

- I don't like to waste time so if I can do two or three things at once without any downside, I will do those things at the same time.

- Working on different ideas that didn't overlap meant the feedback my body gave me was clearer and I could better link any changes to my health/pain to whatever I was doing. For example, if I had changed my diet and my exercises at the same time, I wouldn't have known if it was the food or the exercise which was improving or worsening my pain.

My approach wasn't formalised, I just got started with tackling these three areas of my life – my mind, my body, and my support system. As you read this book, you might be wondering where do you start? What are you capable of?

This is how I would recommend approaching this, knowing what I know now. Sit down with a pad of paper and pen, and draw up a table with three columns. Give those columns the headings of YOUR MIND, YOUR BODY, and YOUR SUPPORT:

YOUR MIND	YOUR BODY	YOUR SUPPORT
Conserve energy	You are what you eat	Educate your friends, family and workmates

As you read each section of this book, pick the first strategy that stands out to you and that you want to try, and note them in each column. I have put my first choices in the table as an example. Yours could be different.

At this point you have enough to get started . . . you don't have to think about what to do next. Just focus on the three choices you have made, and try them until you are satisfied you have completed any one of them. Once you feel you have completed one properly, pick the next strategy you'd like to try from that same group and keep moving forward. This means you're always focusing on three strategies at most at a time, and only ever one strategy from each area at a time.

For example, if you feel you have completed the first strategy in the YOUR SUPPORT column, 'Educate your friends, family and workmates', you might decide to move onto trying 'Find the right support group' next. You can start on that second support strategy, even while you are still working on whatever your first choices were for YOUR MIND and YOUR BODY.

And you keep doing this until you're done . . . whether you beat your arthritis, or it beats you.

A few last thoughts:

- We're only human. You don't have to work on all three strategies all the time every day. On good days you might tackle a bit of each of them or a bigger chunk of one of them. And on bad days, well, you might just take a day off and rest without focusing on any strategy at all. Just make sure you don't go backwards – for example, if you are working on 'You are what you eat' and you're having a bad day, don't go back to eating comfort foods that you've discovered make you feel worse. Instead, find new comfort foods that your body responds well to.

- It's important you don't move on from one strategy to another in any group unless you have done that strategy properly. I believe unlocking your health from arthritis is like a combination lock rather than a padlock – you're looking for the right series of things instead of one simple key. And if you are looking for a series of things that, once combined, unlocks your health, you need to make sure whatever you try is done properly. Otherwise, the progress you've made could be undone (like pulling the wrong block on a precariously stacked Jenga game), or life might just force you back again to do it properly (like building a house without proper foundations, and having rebuild when the cracks in the walls become too many). In either case, the more you do, the worse it can get. Better to avoid that by making sure you're honest with yourself and complete any idea/strategy properly before moving onto another one.

- If you're not sure what you want to start with, and you don't want to start in the same way I did, throw some darts at the list and let fate decide. It doesn't really matter what you start with anyway, you just have to start doing something. Remember what the philosopher Lao Tzu said: 'The journey of a thousand miles must begin with a single step.'

Your Mind

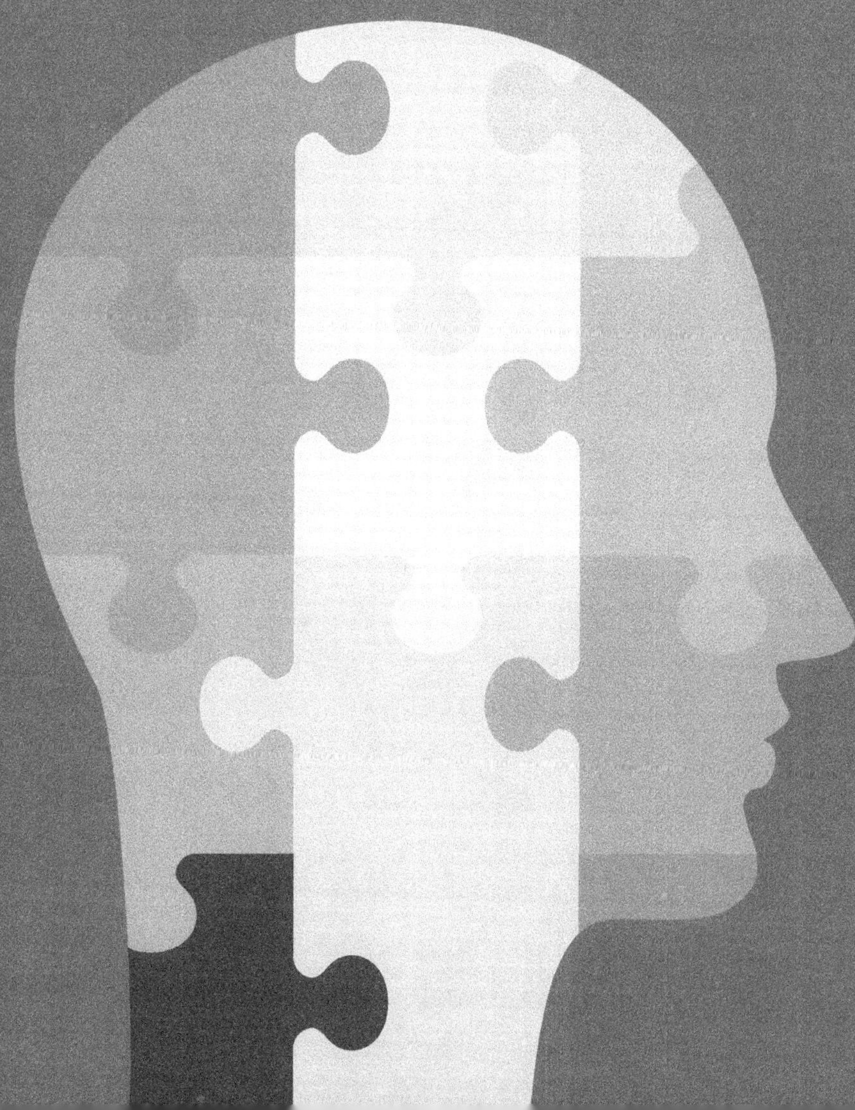

Conserve energy

After living with pain for a while, it became abundantly clear to me that I could no longer count on a good night's sleep to give me enough energy to get through the next day. The pain I was having to manage every day and night was literally sucking the life out of me.

If I was going to fight this properly, I needed as much energy as I could get.

That meant gaining whatever energy I could while resting and recovering AND reducing the leakage of my energy during the days (and nights) as much as possible.

To reduce my energy leakage, I decided I had to remove as much stress from my everyday life, no matter how big or small it might be. Every little bit counted.

To get enough energy to get through a day and hopefully take another step closer to one day being without arthritis, I also had to get the biggest bang for my buck by focusing on removing the easiest things I could that annoyed or stressed me out the most; i.e., I had to deal with those things that required little effort for the biggest results.

So, I started with the smaller annoying things (I call them 'mosquitos' because they're also small and annoying, and suck blood like the stressors sucked my energy) that were easy and quick to deal with:

- I shifted all my pain management tools and medications to the same location in my house, so I didn't have to waste time and energy finding them when I wanted them. It goes without saying you must make sure you put things back in that same place, cupboard or drawer when you're done with them so they're there again when you need them. It's also important that no one else borrow them so they're always there when you need them. You can't be sure when the next pain spike will hit.

- I saw a podiatrist to evaluate how my body walked, and I purchased some personalised orthotics along with better footwear to help me walk a bit easier and take some of the pressure off my knees and ankles.

- I negotiated more flexible starting and ending times with my boss to allow me to work more easily around those times/days when my pain might be worse and I was less able to focus. That way, he trusted me to get the work done and I was less worried about being fired for not finishing work on time or to a high standard because my arthritis had gotten in the way.

It didn't matter how small the mosquitos were. It may feel insignificant changing one small thing, but resolving each one gave me just that little bit more energy that I didn't have to waste anymore. And removing multiple small annoyances can compound if they happen to be related, so the overall effect can be exponentially larger than the energy gained from each individual problem removed separately, added together.

In my effort to reduce stress, no stone was left unturned. As I removed the smaller mosquitos in my life, I worked through larger and larger annoyances that required more effort. And instead of sorting one large problem out in a day (as was possible for the smaller ones), I would take small bites out of larger ones consistently each day to ultimately deal with them.

I didn't care how big the stressors were. And I didn't care how hard they might be to remove properly. I focused on living my life as stress-free as possible so I would have more energy to fight my arthritis.

As I chewed through the things I knew that annoyed me in my life, I also started turning my attention to things that might be stressing me out subconsciously – cannibalising my energy without me knowing. For example, I reached out and connected with my birth father (he left me when I was a baby) just in case I was wasting energy subconsciously worrying about not knowing him.

To help me find these things (because if they were subconscious, I wouldn't be immediately aware of them), I looked at them from other people's points of view. For example, with me not knowing my birth father, I knew many people struggle to live their lives not knowing their parents, and when reconnected they find greater peace in knowing more about their past, where they come from and who they are. And while this felt like poppycock to me (because I believe I don't need to know where I come from to know where I am going), as I said before, I wasn't going to leave any stone unturned . . . which meant I couldn't let my own ego get in my way.

By reducing the stress in my life, I was able to:

- Improve the energy I had on a daily basis.
- Reduce the times I needed to stop and rest.

- Reduce my reliance on others and medicine (which was important for me and the independence I valued).

All of which allowed me to fight harder and longer than may have been the case if my pain spikes had been more frequent, longer or higher as a result of living with less energy.

Focus on positives not negatives

One of the things my specialists told me I should do to help manage my arthritis was to keep a pain diary: a record of my pain levels on a daily or hourly basis, along with a record of the food and drink I was consuming, the rest and sleep I was having, the medications I took, and any physical activities I was doing.

The idea of a pain diary is to identify triggers that increase or reduce pain levels. By identifying the things that might escalate your pain, you can then remove those things to reduce pain naturally. Alternatively, if you can identify things that reduce pain, you can then add more of those on a more regular basis to, again, reduce pain naturally.

Seemed sensible enough.

Unfortunately, this is one of those things that sounds sensible to anyone who has never had to do it.

As someone who has kept a pain diary, I say, 'Don't do it!' Run, Forrest, run!

After a few months of keeping a pain diary, I realised it was training my mind and body to look for any pain in my body regardless of how big or small that pain was. I found this to be very negative and unhelpful as it was forcing me to focus in on the experience of pain, when I really wanted to focus on finding a way to beat my arthritis and no longer be in pain.

Having realised that focusing on the negative can only lead to poor outcomes, I made the drastic decision to burn my pain diary (symbolically cleansing me of the poison the idea created), and I flipped the idea upside down and started keeping a health diary instead. Where before I was recording my pain levels on an hourly or daily basis, now I started recording my without-pain levels instead; i.e., focusing on how well I was rather than how sore I was.

This had two benefits for me:

- It was more positive focusing; i.e., I was looking for a life without pain.

- I was able to use this as a guide to help me reach my goal.

When you don't know how to get what you want (i.e., beat your arthritis), you have to focus on something you can see that links to what you want, to help work out if you're doing the right thing or not.

In my case, beating my arthritis meant being able to live my life with no pain. So even if I (or the specialists) didn't know how to do that, I knew that to achieve a goal of no arthritis, I was probably heading in the right direction if I did things that reduced the pain levels I had to endure. And I was probably heading in the wrong direction if my pain levels increased.

The thing is, you get what you focus on. So, whether you focus on reducing pain or not increasing pain, your brain focuses on pain. If you want to live pain-free, then you must focus on increasing – or not decreasing – your 'pain-free-ness'.

Let me be 100% clear, because this is important – reducing pain is NOT the same as increasing pain-free-ness. I know some of you may look at this and think, 'What you talkin' 'bout, Willis?', but small changes in perspective can result in a huge changes in outcome.

For example, you don't snowboard through trees by avoiding the trees; you snowboard through trees by aiming for the gaps.[1] Even though, logically, thinking 'don't hit the trees' should result in the same outcome as 'aim for the gaps', it won't. Try it yourself one day if you get the chance – 'don't hit the trees' will result in your hitting the trees. 'Aim for the gaps' will result in your snowboarding safely through.

So, I believe it's critical you don't record your pain to help guide you. You record your pain-free-ness (your health) instead. And instead of looking for things you do or eat which increase or decrease pain, you now look for things you do or eat that increase pain-free-ness (health). Small change; big outcome!

Something to bear in mind, though: it is true that when arthritis is no longer active in your body, you will no longer

---

1 Before I became arthritic, I went snowboarding in Whistler, Canada, on a guided lesson. The guide took us off trail and introduced us to a grove of trees, stopping us before we attempted to go through them. He asked us this question: 'How do you snowboard through trees?' Someone offered what seemed like the obvious answer: 'Don't hit the trees.' The guide said, 'You'd think so, right? But that's not right. You need to aim for the gaps. If you aim to not hit the trees, you will hit the trees.' And with that advice, he told us to go through the trees. I mentally told myself, 'Aim for the gaps . . . aim for the gaps . . . aim for the gaps,' but as I got closer to the first tree in front of me, I remember switching and telling myself, 'Don't hit the tree,' and, you guessed it, I hit the tree, faceplanting into a pile of powder at the base. Lesson learned – it didn't happen again, and it's become a useful way to change my perspective on other things.

have to endure pain 24/7. Therefore, increasing pain-free-ness (health) must get you closer to living without arthritis.

It is also true that while you experience pain 24/7 when you are arthritic, it is not 100% true you are not arthritic if you no longer experience pain – it is possible to have no pain and still be arthritic (but this is not common because being pain-free while still arthritic never lasts). If you live with arthritis, whether you still have arthritis or not isn't really important. What is most important is how much pain you live with (or don't have to live with) every day. If I hadn't beaten my arthritis, I would have gladly accepted being pain-free with arthritis. Being without pain, with or without arthritis, is bliss!

So think of your wellness (pain-free-ness) like a Geiger counter that measures radiation – you may not know where the radiation is (because you can't see it), but if the Geiger counter pings faster then you're heading closer to the radiation source. If the Geiger counter pings slower, then you're moving away from it. As your pain-free-ness increases, you are moving closer to your goal. As your pain-free-ness decreases, you're moving further away from where you want to be.

Using a health diary won't in itself cure you, but it will help you stay on the right path towards living without arthritis – as long as you're paying attention to your body and being honest with yourself.

Don't be a victim

Pre-arthritis, I read about Carolyn Myss's[2] theory of *woundology*. Her theory was that some people don't heal because they've made an identity out of woundedness. They like the attention it gets them and don't want to give it up.

If you want to beat your arthritis, you need to make sure you do not let yourself milk people's support when you don't really need it, just because it makes you feel good. The goal is to live without arthritis . . . not use it to get people's sympathy.

So I cannot say this strongly enough: do not let your arthritis define you!

---

2 Carolyn Myss has written many wonderful books; I found *Why People Don't Heal and How They Can* (Sydney: Bantam Books, 1997) and *Sacred Contracts* (Sydney: Bantam Books, 2002) particularly useful.

Do not use your arthritis as an excuse to get people's sympathy and support!

And do not let arthritis be your life!

Yes, it sucks to live in pain 24/7, never knowing from hour to hour whether the pain you have to endure will be a mild 3 out of 10, or a debilitating 9 out of 10.

It can be easy to start believing 'woe is me' or 'this is my life forever' (particularly on bad days when you are at your weakest). Hell, there were times my mind started to run off imagining a future of 24/7 pain till death do I part.

But the arthritis I endured was not me. It was just a part of my life. And even though I didn't know how I got it, I accepted that somehow I was responsible for getting arthritis by way of my life choices. Ignorance is no defence.

I owned my arthritis – lock, stock and barrel. I didn't want it . . . true. But I had it. No one else caused it or gave it to me. It was mine.

This was also my life and no one else's. And even though my doctor and specialists told me I'd live with my arthritis forever, they were not me. This was my life, not theirs. And I wasn't about to let them tell me how I was going to live it.

So while you have to endure your arthritis like I did, do not let it take over your life. The moment you do that, you give your arthritis control, and I guarantee you will never cure yourself if you rely on your arthritis to get you sympathy and attention from others. Hold onto the vision of being the victor . . . and not the victim.

Focus on what you can control – not what you can't

When you have arthritis, it's easy to feel like your life is out of your control.

Having arthritis means you won't be able to do some of the things you used to anymore, either because it might be unsafe due to you having less coordination or strength, or because you're in too much pain (or you know you'll end up in a lot of pain afterwards).

And because we're human, we initially only see that which we cannot do anymore; we lose sight of what we can still do, and the new things we could start doing are completely invisible to us.

As Helen Keller once said, 'When one door of happiness closes, another opens; but often we look so long at the closed door that we do not see the one which has been opened for us.'

Yes, arthritis sucks. But focusing on everything you can't do anymore due to arthritis sucks even more.

I know that me telling you to get over it won't help. We all need however long it takes to get over ourselves and what we see we've lost.

It took me six months to get past denying I had arthritis AND my anger that I had lost my ability to do any of the physical activities I enjoyed due to the fear of, or actually getting, pain.

How long it will take you is like asking 'how long is a piece of string?' It could take more time; it could take less.

But I know with 100% certainty, if you don't find a way to stop focusing on what you can't do anymore, and what you've lost, you won't move one step closer to being free from arthritis.

I don't recall exactly how I moved past what I lost and what I couldn't do anymore. I suspect in hindsight my change came from a number of things:

- Realising that focusing on a problem that I didn't know how to solve was a waste of my time and energy – and as I talked about earlier, it was extremely important to me to have and conserve as much energy as I could to help me 'fight' this.

- Focusing on what I couldn't do distracted me from focusing on my vision of living without arthritis. If I wanted to achieve my vision of being arthritis-free, I'd have to stop looking at what I couldn't do and start focusing on what I could do instead.

- I started asking if I couldn't do my rollerblading, weight lifting, kayaking, dancing, snowboarding, biking . . . then maybe I could find alternatives I could do instead. Maybe I could find some new physical activities I had never done that I could enjoy? Or maybe I could change how I biked, or how I lifted weights in ways that still allowed me to do the things I enjoyed while minimising the risk of pain?

- Finding ways to do the things I couldn't with no risk of pain. I am a gamer – I like to play games on my computer – so I used my games to experience things I struggled with in real life while arthritic. For example, I couldn't snowboard anymore so I used to play snowboarding games to remember what it felt like carving a line down a mountain in the fresh powder. I also used computer games to distract me from my pain and life at times – games where I could jump, run and kill bad guys to save the world (things I couldn't do in real life either, due to my arthritis . . . or because they were totally socially unacceptable).

- Being grateful for what I had. I had a partner who loved me and whom I loved. I could still get to and from work without help. I would have days with only 3 out of 10 pain and on those days I could pretty much do anything. I had a job that I could go to and keep earning income to help fund my personal war on arthritis. I had friends, family and workmates who understood what I was having to deal with and were there if I asked.

Ultimately, I believe the quickest way you can stop focusing on what you've lost and what you can't do anymore is by doing a combination of the following three things:

- Let it all out and do whatever works for you to release all that pain, frustration, regret, anger . . . everything that's holding you back. Try:
    - punching the crap out of a punching bag – just make sure you do this in a way that doesn't flare up your pain or injure your joints.

- screaming into a pillow. I admit this can feel embarrassing, but who really cares if you're by yourself when you do it?

- go to one of those 'wrecking rooms' where you suit up in protective clothing and are allowed to smash various objects with a baseball bat, or throw glass/crockery across the room (you could do that in your own home, but you'll have a mess to clean up afterwards . . . plus you don't want to risk getting shards of glass/crockery in your eye). These weren't around when I was battling my arthritis, but if they were, I would have definitely used them.

You might have to do this daily, weekly or just as needed until you've exhausted all the thoughts you have of what you can't do anymore. The idea is to help shift your focus over time so initially there might be frequent shouting/yelling/punching/smashing, but hopefully you will find that gradually reducing over time.

- Be grateful for what you have. You're alive! Others are less fortunate – there are people who died younger than you and never got to experience all that life can offer. Maybe you want to see your child grow up and be everything they want to be.

Maybe you haven't fallen in love yet – you can't do that dead. Maybe someone loves you . . . despite your pain with arthritis.

There is a lot to be grateful for . . . but only if you know how lucky you are. And believe me when I tell you this: if you live in a country where you have running water (hot and cold), reliable power and internet, a roof over your head, and access to food, you can start with being grateful for those – because there are many people in this world who don't have them.

If you aren't used to being grateful for what you do have (probably because, like most humans, we instead covet what we don't have), then this is a good opportunity to start learning how to be grateful. It won't only be helpful with you dealing with your arthritis, but being grateful also helps with being more understanding of others who may not have some of the things you might have or have access to. And this world can always do with more understanding of others.

If being grateful is something you're unfamiliar with then start small. Pick something that made you smile today and be grateful for whatever that was. Maybe it was a stranger who smiled at you; maybe it was nature putting on a show somehow (like recently, I saw a magpie divebombing a hawk and it made me smile . . . that magpie had some kind of F-U attitude to take on a hawk and I admire that type of attitude).

- Find ways to do the things you love. This will remind you that life is precious and valuable (and not black and horrible due to arthritis).

Maybe you have things you want to do before you do eventually pass away (a bucket list)? Why not do them while you still can? Smell that rose. Pat that dog. Love your partner and your children. Savour that food. Do something to make someone you care about smile. Hell, do something to make a stranger smile.

Focus on what's most important to you – something you would live and die for. And get better at removing/dismissing anything that doesn't contribute to whatever is most important to you. If you're lucky, you already know what is most important to you and you've built that into your life. Making space in your life every day for whatever is most important to you – whether that's you actually doing it, or moving closer to it – will always fill you with passion and LIFE. And that's a good thing. As is getting rid of everything from your life that distracts you from that.

If you don't know what is most important to you, well, maybe now is a good time to reflect on where you are and work that out for yourself. It must be yours and not someone else's, and definitely not what others tell you should be most important to you, and you can build it into your life moving forward. For me, it was the need to leave the world a better place than when I came into it, and I'm doing that via my business, using a goal of 'building better worlds through better business'. Being of service to others is what I live for. This book is one way I can build a better world by providing some hope to other arthritis sufferers that there *is* hope – despite what specialists and doctors may say.

Live for now – do not let your mind wander into unwanted futures

In the three years I fought my arthritis, I remember catching my mind wandering too far into the future maybe once or twice.

Thanks to the philosophy I'd studied pre-arthritis, I was pretty good at living 'now' and not thinking too much into my future.

However, I am human, and I recall one day when I let my guard down and let my mind wander further than it needed to. My guess now is that I was probably hungry, tired, and having a bad pain day – a bad combination that distracted me from keeping my mind away from ruminating about an unknown future (particularly a depressing one like living in pain forever).

So, on this particular day I remember my mind wandered into my future with arthritis (not without). This was years into the future, and I remember carrying the weight of all that time and the pain I endured over those years yet to come. For me, it wasn't just that decades from then I was still arthritic, it was more I had lived and experienced every day between now and then and the pain over that entire time.

It sucked. It sucked a lot.

I felt the pain and suffering I had endured over those years and decades well up inside me and start to wash over me. I felt the things I couldn't and didn't do over that time. I felt the discomfort from the realisation my life was dictated by this. I felt the lack of power I had over whatever was my life past that point in the future.

I also remember the feeling of sadness grabbing at me, trying to pull me down. I could feel the tears for everything I had lost welling up inside every cell in my body . . . as well as in my eyes.

And as this was happening, I also recall a distinct moment of clarity; a thought asking, 'What the fuck are you doing?'

I realised I had let my mind wander off to consider a future I wasn't aiming for – a future I didn't want, a future that wasn't real, a future that may never happen – and I was losing my grip on reality today as a result.

I was being stupid and, dare I say it, delusional.

I had forgotten who I was, where I was, and what I was living for today. I was ignoring what I was fighting for (a life without pain). I had also forgotten everything I had done so far and the smaller battles I had won (like the success I'd had with some dietary changes).

I remember quickly telling myself off for being so stupid and getting upset over things that hadn't happened (and would never happen if I got my way).

And I quickly 'reset' my thinking to return to 'now' and where I was.

Since then, I have never let my mind do that again. I can't tell you what would have happened if that imaginary future had enveloped me – if that sadness of all the pain I endured up to that moment had been allowed to wash over me completely. To be honest, it scares me to think what would have happened because it was so fast and strong and dark that I know it could have easily washed me away to a place that I may have never returned from . . . so for me it's better to never get there in the first place. I thank whatever spirit (whether inner or outer) that jumped to my attention at the time to 'wake me up'.

If you don't have the inner strength to face whatever demons may arise in your journey, build 'safety nets' (friends, family, support groups, mind tricks you may already have) around you that you can rely on when those moments arise. Because you are human, you will face dark days where it hurts to go on, where you doubt yourself, where you lose sight of the possibility you might beat your arthritis, where you believe everyone else and forget about those (unfortunately rare) cases of people who have beaten it . . . and where you question what's the point.

If you feel that dark grey cloud of despair rising, do whatever works for you to stand against it and remain focused on now, today, and everything you have done . . . and use the light of knowing if one person can beat their arthritis (like I did), then it's possible others can too.

Whatever happens in your case, I cannot reinforce enough to make sure you don't dwell on uncertain futures – other than one where you too may find your way through this to live free of arthritis.

Learn from the wisdom of others before you

Part of my journey included exploring philosophies and religions from around the world to help me better understand what may be going on. The idea being that improving my understanding of the world, the universe and society might ultimately highlight better choices and hopefully better outcomes in my life in general.

I had an interest in Western philosophies and religions before I became arthritic, particularly the work of Marcus Aurelius, Shane Mulhall, Robert A. Johnson, Robert Bly, and Carl Jung. I expanded that knowledge while I was arthritic by attending practical philosophy classes offered by the School of Philosophy in Auckland, learning more about happiness, love, and freedom.

While I had learned a lot from Western philosophy and religion, there was something about Eastern philosophy that intrigued me, and so I started to explore the Bhagavad Gita, the teachings of the Dalai Lama, and the work of Bruce Lee, who had been heavily influenced by Taoism and Buddhism. I suspected that as Eastern philosophies were older, they had more experience/wisdom/history to offer, and I believe there is a lot of truth to be learned from ancient wisdom.

The message I was getting from Western medicine was pretty clear cut – live with arthritis for life with progressively stronger pain meds (and hope/pray Western science finds a cure – bearing in mind arthritis itself will not kill you, so finding a cure is not high on the to-do list in medicine). But when I started exploring Eastern philosophies, I uncovered one specific idea that I found both interesting and helpful – yin and yang. In ancient Chinese philosophy, yin and yang is a concept of dualism, describing how seemingly opposite or contrary forces may actually be complementary, interconnected, and interdependent in the natural world, and how they may give rise to each other as they interrelate.

This is in direct opposition to the Western idea of balance which is more like a seesaw, with opposite or contrary forces on either side in a binary relationship (one or the other). Think about the Western idea of work/life balance and how 'conventional' wisdom requires you to trade one off for the other (which I believe is complete nonsense because work/ life is not binary).

Applying yin and yang to work/life accepts that work and life complement each other, are interconnected and inter-dependent. The same applies to hot and cold . . . light and dark . . . and also sickness and health.

And here's where I found a very interesting quote that clarified how health and sickness balance each other in yin and yang: 'The seeds of sickness are found in health, just as the seeds of health are found in sickness.'[3]

I have to say this specific quote hit me like a freight train at the time, and it has stuck with me ever since. I suspect it will be one of the final things that fades from my brain on my eventual death bed. It was like someone had shined a black light on the inside of my brain and I could now see so much more than what I already thought I knew . . . all previously hidden from my view.

I think the reason this particular quote made perfect sense to me was because I had worked out while growing up with the advent of the internet and Google that the answer to any question was contained in the question; i.e., you have

---

3 This quote came from a book I read decades ago now. Unfortunately I never wrote down the book's title or the author's name, and I haven't been able to find the source again.

to ask the right question to get the right answer. Ask the wrong question and you won't find the answer you're looking for.

I wasn't 100% clear how it happened, but reflecting on my life pre-arthritis with yin and yang as a filter suggested that the seeds of my arthritis must have been contained in the life I'd been living. My arthritis 'grew' from the apparently 'healthy' lifestyle I led.

While uncovering what I had done to turn my arthritis on was an interesting puzzle to solve (so I could turn it off), I was more interested in the idea that yin and yang offered that I might be able to find the 'seeds of health' within my arthritis that I could feed to move away from being arthritic.

So I now had two different ways of healing myself – both related to each other:

1. If my arthritis could be turned on then it could be turned off . . . if I could find the switch and reset it.

2. I could become healthy again by essentially feeding my health and starving my sickness – all I had to do was to find the 'seeds of health' within my arthritis.

Now I get it – this is vague as hell and on the face of it very unhelpful if you want out from arthritis. How the hell are you supposed to turn off your arthritis when you're not sure what your switch is? And how are you supposed to feed the 'seeds of health' in your arthritis when you don't know what they are for you?

All I can say is . . . think of this like a big jigsaw puzzle where you don't have the box to guide you, in which case any hint or clue is better than nothing.

Before reading this, you were probably looking for one thing – a cure. What I'm sharing in this section is that there are two possible cures – find whatever switch that flicked on to activate your arthritis and turn it back off, or work out the 'seeds of health' within your arthritis to feed so you effectively starve your arthritis to death.

Remember that I had nothing to guide me. I had to do this pretty much by myself, in the dark, with a blindfold, with my hands tied behind my back. You at least have the bread-crumbs I used to help find my way back again. And that's better than what I started with.

Psychologists and counsellors

You might have heard the phrase 'you are what you eat'. Some people interpret this literally, that our bodies are the result of what we put in our mouths. Eat junk food . . . get a junk body.

But considering it philosophically, its meaning is much wider than just the literal food we eat and its effect on our body. Its wider meaning encompasses everything we take into our bodies – not just food, but also the music we listen to, the books we read, the movies and television we watch, and all the thoughts, smells, and experiences we might have.

And just as our bodies might react poorly if we eat bad food, our bodies can also react badly to accepting bad thoughts, experiences, music, books, movies, etc.

This means if we are what we eat, and eating good food leads to a good body, then it must also be true that if our body is not working properly in some way (e.g., experiencing arthritis), it is possible we've made poor choices in what we 'ate' which manifested in our bodies as whatever problems we're now experiencing.

The problem is how to work out what's good and bad for you after the fact, especially if the link isn't obvious. How do you know if a certain idea or belief you live with may be contributing to an ulcer, a twitch, your arthritis, or some other annoying health problem? How do you know which foods you should continue to eat, and which foods you should stop so they don't keep contributing to your malfunctioning body?

Not only that, but how do you look for something when you do not know what you are looking for? As humans, we're good at ignoring that which we don't understand. We have blind spots where we can't see things that might be right in front of us. We have biases we look for and reinforce towards things we like and want to be true, and away from things we don't like and don't want to be true.

This is where you need someone else to help you. Someone who understands the human brain. Someone who is objective and can hear and see things you may be ignoring. Someone who can unpack your way of thinking and your beliefs, and how these could be helping or hindering your life. Someone like a counsellor or psychologist.

So, I went looking for a counsellor to do just that.

Full transparency . . . before I experienced arthritis, I didn't believe in counselling. I thought that sitting with someone and talking about your shit until you say something you think might be the answer was a waste of time. I have always been the sort of guy that thinks through whatever is going wrong and reworks the problem or situation until it's not wrong anymore (more do . . . less talk).

However, as I mentioned before, if I wanted to get rid of my arthritis, no stone could be left unturned. No option could be left untried. Being uncomfortable wasn't allowed to be an excuse to avoid doing something that might help. Being in pain 24/7 was more uncomfortable than subjecting myself to a counsellor.

So, I started seeing a counsellor once every three weeks to talk about anything that 'came up'.

To avoid wasting the consultations talking about life in general (counsellors aren't cheap), I set up a framework with my counsellor for our consultations to focus on pain and things that might be contributing to it manifesting in my body as arthritis.

I also gave her full power to call me on any BS I might try to deflect or avoid anything that came up in our sessions, and in return I promised I would not get upset if she called me on any BS. I've read a lot about human behaviour, counselling, and psychology so I know a lot of the 'tricks' which also means I know how to deflect, avoid, or say the right things to move things along.

So, with her help, over the course of four months (interestingly enough, the months leading up to my arthritis going away), we picked away at my life. We discussed things like:

- The difference between existing versus living.
- My being a perfectionist and being self-critical, my fear of failure/embarrassment and how I am bad at forgiving myself for failings, and my overall self-personal worth.
- Why I am so hard on myself; why I push myself.
- My relationship history and how I struggle with connecting with others.
- My tendency towards addiction, expressed via gaming or devouring information on specific topics of interest to the nth degree – addictions which could be used to repress rage/anger.

- My family background/childhood history – did I see my mum break up with my birth dad as an infant? Was I carrying that stress still?

- Trying to understand balance; finding the willingness to change.

- Music/dream therapy and interpretation of dreams.

- The conflict between my internal and external worlds, particularly between creativity and perfectionism.

- How I internalised anger/rage, and my preference to hurt myself rather than risk others by sharing/expressing 'negative' emotions.

Yes, sometimes I felt stupid in my sessions – music/dream therapy was the worst for me. Sometimes things made absolutely no sense to me (music therapy again). But if I got new angles about myself, my arthritis, and my pain, then it was all worth it.

And regardless of what came from each session or how I felt about it, I dug in and I did the work – I read relevant books, explored the internet, and pushed myself and my boundaries to test my limitations. I reflected on everything I digested and experienced from new perspectives, building on what I had already tried where relevant, and then I would share that in the next session with my counsellor.

Doing this helped me to find my blind spots – those things I couldn't see . . . or those things I might have been ignoring and dismissing prematurely. For example, with the issue of my birth father leaving me when I was an infant. On the advice of my counsellor, I talked with my mum to hear her perspective and better understand what had been going on at the time, and I let my birth father into my life. He had been trying to see me for a few years, but I had rejected his invitations because I considered my stepdad to be my dad – he was the man who raised me as his son. I had a dad already and I believed I didn't need to look back to move forward. Even though I hadn't consciously have any problems with my birth father not being in my life, meeting up with him did give me some resolution, and I could say that it was an issue I explored fully in my quest.

If you do decide to add a counsellor or psychologist to your arsenal against arthritis, I believe you need to be very clear about what you hope to achieve with them – and make sure you tell them this. I also believe you need to pick the right counsellor for you. My recommendations would be:

- Pick someone who is different to you in as many ways as possible. For example, if you are male, pick a female counsellor; if you're a female, pick a male – you'll get a perspective you are less familiar with (there's a reason most men don't understand women, and vice versa).

- Pick someone older and more experienced – they are more likely to call you on any BS you might try. Younger, less experienced counsellors might not want to risk losing you as a client so might be less likely to confront you on any BS.

- Pick someone who has experience working with people in pain. If you want to live a life without pain, then you must work with someone who understands the experience of pain in its various forms – that way you have a better chance of gaining insights into thoughts that might manifest as pain in your body and contribute to or reduce pain.

- As the Buddhist teacher Pema Chödrön wrote, 'Fear is a natural reaction to moving closer to the truth.'[4] Pick someone who makes you a little bit anxious and/or uncomfortable because they're digging deep and pushing you in the right direction – just make sure you're not too uncomfortable (you must work together after all).

---

4 Pema Chödrön, *When Things Fall Apart: Heart Advice for Difficult Times* (Boston: Shambhala Publications, 1997), 2.

And keep an open mind. Doing things that are different, or that make you uncomfortable might unlock the last piece of the combination for turning off your arthritis. You never know.

One last thing . . . even after my arthritis was gone physically, I continued meeting with my counsellor for another two years on a less regular basis, stopping only when I no longer felt anxious or uncomfortable seeing them. And while I still hadn't fully unpacked the baggage I had picked up while being arthritic, or from my life before, I was comfortable enough with myself by that point that I no longer needed to understand why I did or thought certain things.

I still never got music therapy . . . but I'm okay with that.

Shadow work

While working with my counsellor, we touched on a theory about the human psyche called the 'shadow'. This concept was coined by the Swiss psychiatrist Carl Jung in the early 20th century as one of the four archetypes explaining unconscious and subconscious human thought and behaviour.

Simply put, the shadow is made up of the part of ourselves that we hide from everyone . . . including from ourselves. It is every part of us we don't want to acknowledge about ourselves or allow society to see, so we repress them, pushing them deep into our unconscious psyche. The shadow includes things that might be a source of shame or anxiety, or things that don't fit into dominant social attitudes, like:

- Regrets or shameful experiences.

- Our fears.

- Taboo mental images or thoughts.
- Socially or personally unacceptable sexual desires.
- Emotions like envy, greed or anger.
- Perceived weaknesses.

We all have these things. Things we do not want to admit to ourselves or others. And rather than confront the things we don't like about ourselves, our brain does a clever trick and pretends they do not exist. And we do that by locking these parts of us away in the darkest and deepest part of consciousness to ensure they never see the light of day. And we do this because we believe, if allowed to surface, these parts of us would put our very existence in society and with others at risk.

However, if you have ever played with a beach ball in a pool, you will know what happens if you try to push it down and keep it under the water. No matter how hard you try, sooner or later that beach ball is going to pop up to the surface. In fact, the harder you push that ball under, the deeper you push that ball down, the harder it will fight to get to the surface.

And so it is also with the shadow. Despite relegating the worst of ourselves to the deepest and darkest corner of our subconscious, our shadow constantly leaks back into our conscious lives through our dreams (or nightmares) and when we're at our weakest (like when we're tired, hungry, or stressed out), no doubt surprising both ourselves and others who may be around us at the time.

Suppressing one's true self (including the shadow part of ourselves we do not like) cannot be healthy. Keeping the shadow parts of us away from the light of day requires energy, and as far as I was concerned, it was energy better spent managing my pain and arthritis.

And so it was that I decided I wanted to face my shadow to better understand myself and reduce the amount of energy I was no doubt wasting subconsciously to repress those parts of me.

First, it is important to note that facing one's shadow is incredibly difficult because it's scary. As mentioned before, our brain pretends those parts of us don't exist . . . which means they're not easy to find. And even if or when you do find them, they're not in daylight; they're hidden in the darkest part of ourselves, and you are instinctively afraid of them as you get closer to them (which incidentally is a good guide to work out if you're getting close to any shadow part of yourself).

If you're not prepared to be honest with yourself, you will struggle facing your shadow. The goal isn't to cure your shadow. Your goal is to have a relationship with your shadow; to be aware of the things you think rather than run and hide from them. Let it live in daylight. Make the subconscious conscious. This doesn't mean you live your shadow thoughts – just recognise they are just thoughts, and you can accept them as such without having to act on them.

With the help of my counsellor, I started poking around my shadow and uncovered something I think is really interesting. Our shadow contains wisdom. Things can be scary because we don't see them for what they really are. We might fear the greatness of realising whatever we are supressing – that is, our greatest strength can hurt as much as it can help. If we only see how much we could hurt someone with our greatest strength, then it becomes shadow.

For example, one of my greatest strengths is observing more than most people do about any given situation . . . and not being burdened by societal niceties when talking with others (I'm brutally honest – that's the autistic part of me). This has resulted in people getting hurt when I answer some question they wanted my opinion on, because I got too close to some truth about them that they didn't want to hear.

I learned very quickly that people don't really want the truth to questions about themselves; I believe most people ask questions in order to validate their own thoughts. So when I gave my response (based on everything I could see . . . or not see), and it didn't validate what they thought, they got upset. When people get upset over something I say, I get upset too because I don't like hurting people . . . even if it is unintentional. So, to avoid hurting people, and to avoid becoming no-friends-Brydon, I chose to supress telling people what I thought.

The problem with me suppressing honesty for the sake of other people's feelings and possible friendships was that I was lying to myself. Not only that, by being nice and not so honest (under the false justification that I cared about the other person), I knew I wasn't really helping them by telling them what they wanted to hear, rather than what they needed to hear (even if they may not like it).

It wasn't until later years I realised sharing my truths wasn't bad – it was powerful. I just had to learn how to share my observations in ways that didn't hurt others, particularly when my observed truths differed from theirs. I just needed to take responsibility and make the effort to find a way to share my observations in ways that honoured those observations AND still showed I did care AND minimised possible offense to the other (which nowadays starts with the statement, 'Are you sure you want my opinion about "X"?')

I believe it's the same for all aspects of our shadow. Much like yin and yang, we are only seeing one side of any aspect of our shadow (and that's the 'dark' side). It is only by uncovering and then seeking true understanding of that aspect of your shadow will you see the other side (the 'light' side). By doing so, you release that aspect from the darkest recesses of your psyche to share in your life in the light of day.

How you approach your shadow and what you get from that will be unique to you. I know my shadow is not yours, as is the case your shadow is not mine. That means I have no answers for you in this area, other than I believe there is value in better understanding our shadow.

We may never get to see our shadow in its entirety, and we may never really comprehend it completely either. But avoiding it, keeping it hidden, and never understanding it can't be good for our spirit, nor our mind or our body.

I like to think of uncovering your shadow like the Dr Seuss story *What Was I Scared Of?,* where the narrator keeps running into an empty pair of pale green pants. He is terrified of the pants, which stand up and move even though no one is inside them, but soon discovers that the ghostly pants are equally scared of him. From that point on, the fears dissipate and the narrator and the pants become quite good friends.

Your shadow just wants to be understood hence it is always searching for you . . . wanting to 'share' with you. The problem is the shadow is scary to us so we tend to avoid it. It is only once you and your shadow are unable (or unwilling) to run away, and you pay close attention, you realise your shadow might be just as scared of you as you are of it. And once you get past your fear, and you see your shadow for what it really is, or what it could be, you and your shadow might be able to live together without the need to keep it locked away.

There are no tricks to finding or facing your shadow, other than recognising you know you are getting closer to your shadow when you want to turn around, run away, do anything else, feel anxious, or deflect . . . and that is when you need to keep moving in closer. Being curious and seeking better understanding will also help.

Also recognise you are unlikely to never have a shadow – it's not a problem to be solved. I'm still poking around in the darkest regions of who I am to better understand mine, and I probably will be for the rest of my life. I see my shadow as a source of wisdom . . . which it will share with me when I'm ready and willing to accept it.

Your Support

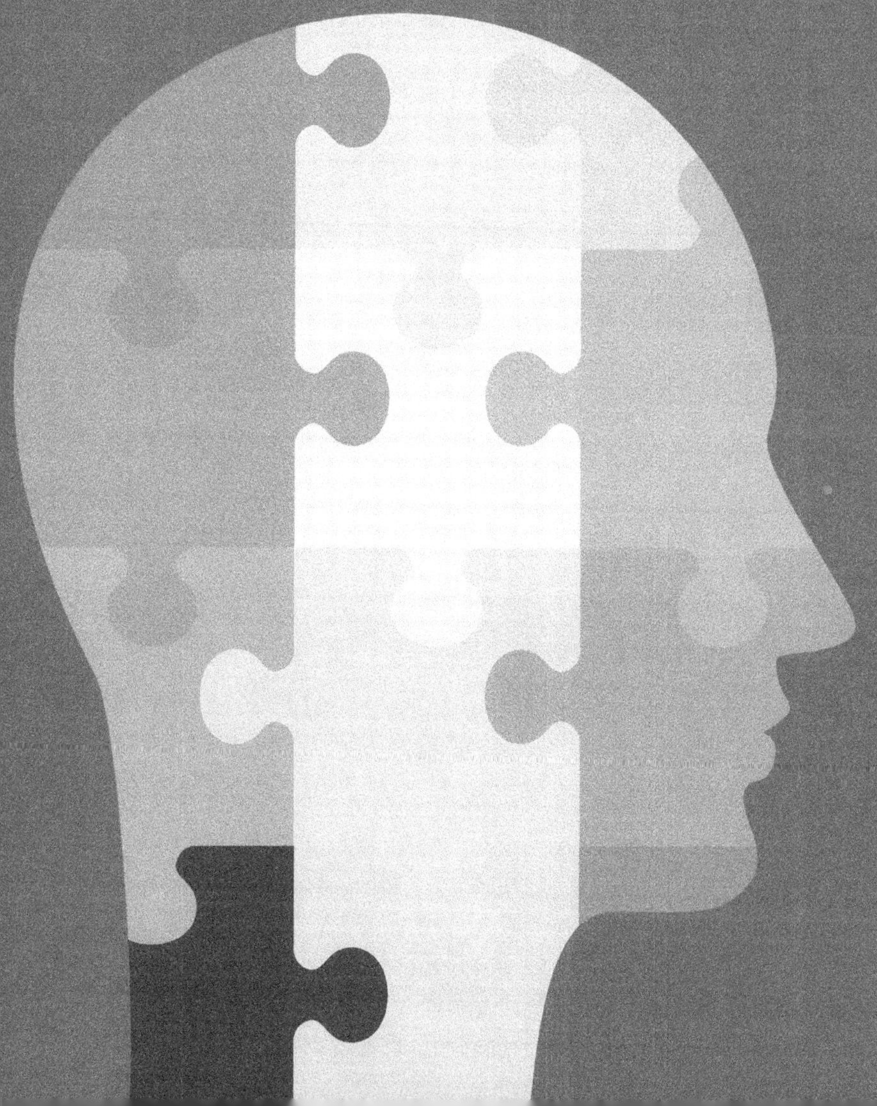

Educate your friends, family and workmates

The myths that surround arthritis annoyed me when it came to the people in my life. It seemed that everyone had a 'story' of arthritis and what it meant to them. It's a pretty common ailment, as it turns out.

Unfortunately, what's not commonly understood is that not all arthritis is the same. And not all experiences of arthritis are the same, either. While living in pain may be a common factor, arthritis is a very unique experience to each individual and those around them.

My story of arthritis was not the same as my friend's grandmother's. It also wasn't the same as another workmate's dad's.

I got tired of managing the egos of people who were well meaning, and having to educate them on my experience (as well as how I was managing it by wanting to cure myself as opposed to living with it, like my friend's grandmother or workmate's dad).

I decided to help explain what arthritis meant to me, and help those around me to better understand what I was dealing with so they didn't make false assumptions about me and my illness. I shared with all my friends and family what I was having to deal with and let them know that I didn't want their sympathy and I didn't want their help unless I asked for it. I chose to do this in groups so I didn't have to explain it to each person separately (which would have been too slow and repetitive for me).

I helped them to better understand that planning for me was difficult because I could never anticipate what level of pain I could have at any time in the future. My pain could be anywhere between 3 out of 10 on good days and 9 out of 10 on bad days, and it was pretty much random.

I wanted them to understand that when I was enduring a pain spike of about 8 out of 10 or more, I might need to leave wherever I was to find a dark and quiet room. And depending on what I had been doing prior to the bad pain spike, and how long it took for that pain spike to pass,

I might or might not be able to rejoin whatever it was I was doing before the pain spike washed over me.

Educating my friends, family and workmates removed any false assumptions they might have had and helped make sure everyone understood my journey better. My friends, family and workmates knew better how to help me. And that in turn helped me not worry about what they may be thinking or feeling, and not have to constantly deal with false assumptions they might make about my illness.

Independence versus support

I am a fiercely independent person. Becoming arthritic challenged my independence. There were times I needed help and support due to my pain that I wouldn't have needed when I was healthy, so asking for help sucked for me!

On my worst days when my pain was circling around 8 or 9 out of 10, it would be hard to hide the pain I was enduring, even though I did my best to not let others see how much pain I was dealing with. I never wanted anyone's sympathy.

For the most part, I hid my pain because of two reasons:

- People would react to my pain in ways I didn't like: some people got sad thinking about the pain I was enduring; others would go out of their way to do things for me, sometimes uninvited or without offering, and sometimes doing things I preferred to do myself even if I was in pain.

- The pain was mine to endure and no one else needed to know or suffer through what I was experiencing, so I was saving them from that.

The problem for me was, while people justified their actions as helping me, they were actually being selfish and helping themselves to minimise their discomfort at seeing me in pain.

While I understood that their intentions were good, if I wanted help I would ask for it. Until then, I was okay doing whatever it was that I was doing . . . even if I was in some pain.

Taking things off me, doing things for me – even though it was more difficult for me than normal – made me feel weak. It robbed me of my independence. It took away the challenge of whatever it was that I was doing while arthritic. And more importantly, I couldn't work out if the strategies I was trying were moving me closer or further away from finding a way to live arthritis-free. Because when someone did something for me that I didn't invite them to do, I didn't get an opportunity to learn from the experience and outcome.

So I had to explain to all my friends, family, and the people I worked with that they should ask if I wanted their help before actually doing anything. That gave me the choice and maintained my independence and dignity. And if they forgot to ask before helping, I promised them I would politely thank them for trying to help and also remind them that I could manage if I didn't need their help at that time. I would also let them know that if I did need their help at any point, they'd be the first to know.

Everyone has their own levels of pain they're willing to endure before accepting help. You may be more willing to ask for or accept help than I was. And I know it can be hard asking for help – particularly as a male – because to do so can be seen as being weak. I also know asking for help can be a sign of strength.

The 'trick', I believe, is knowing your own true limit where you don't ask for or accept help all the time, and at the same time never avoid asking for help when you really do need it. There is a big difference between owning your arthritis and getting help when you really need it, compared to letting your arthritis own you and letting everyone do everything for you (see 'Don't be a victim', p. 29).

Find the right support group

I was told it would be a good idea to join the arthritis support group in my region, seeing as there would be a range of people enduring different types of arthritis in the group, and a wealth of experience and knowledge to be gained from those people. It can be helpful to know you're not alone.

I only ever went to one group meeting because I found the experience too negative for me. For the most part, they accepted their lot in terms of pain and pain meds . . . and I wasn't interested in that. I was going to fight this (with a view to beating it) and being around people who accepted their arthritis for life wasn't helpful.

For me, I think it's more valuable to be around a group who are heading in the same direction as you want to be. There is no doubt you can learn a lot about how to manage arthritis and pain from others facing the same problem. However, you are unlikely to learn more than that if they are only focused on getting through their lives, managing their pain and arthritis as opposed to the possibility of beating it.

And while the support group I went to wasn't of much use for me (apart from me confirming it wasn't going to be useful), I still do recommend that you should try to find one for yourself, if you haven't done so already. You may get more out of a group than I did. You might get a group more focused on curing themselves than just managing their arthritis for life. You never know.

Pain meds – the necessary evil of balancing pain with side effects/dependence

Traditional Western medicine has, as of yet, been unable to cure arthritis. The best it can offer is pain reduction using pain meds – which typically get progressively stronger as your body adapts to them. This means, at this point in time, Western medicine can't solve your problem of being arthritic. It can only deal with some of the symptoms.

I'm more interested in preventing problems than solving them. For example, in this case, I was focused on beating arthritis, more than reducing or removing my pain that came from being arthritic. So from that aspect, pain meds were a concern.

The longer it took me to find a solution to my arthritis, the stronger my pain meds would get. Stronger pain meds meant I faced greater risks from the side effects of the progressively stronger medication, as well as potential dependency issues caused by being on them for long periods of time. I was 'fortunate' to be taking a commonly prescribed nonsteroidal anti-inflammatory painkiller, which has a main side effect of contributing to stomach ulcers. Luckily for me, I didn't develop stomach ulcers while taking this medicine, but I was very aware that it might just be a matter of time before I did. So it was important for me to do whatever I could to prevent or delay that from happening.

So I made two decisions that came with consequences I had to be willing to accept.

1. I would not rely on pain meds all the time. Instead, I would rely on them more on the worse days and use them less on the better days. This would likely mean I would have to endure a bit more pain than if I stayed on the meds all the time. This in turn meant I needed to have a variety of non-medicinal 'tricks' that could help manage pain levels.

2. I would have periods when I would deliberately stay off my meds so I could 'test' how much pain I was having to endure (and how much pain the meds were covering when I was taking them). Think of it this way – if you were on the meds all the time and you stumbled into curing yourself on

whatever path you follow, how would you know if you are no longer arthritic?

The main consequence I faced was having to endure more pain while off the meds than I would have if I kept taking them. Some of the meds I took were slow release, which meant they had to build up in my system before I would feel any benefit from them (think of it like a time lag). That could be tricky if my pain spiked at the high end suddenly – I could be a good 24 hours away from the pain meds doing their job again if I had stopped them for more than 24 hours previously.

However, the benefits for me (which I considered greater than the consequences) were the following:

- Having to face my pain more would give me the opportunity to become mentally and emotionally stronger.
- Enduring more pain would motivate me to find more tricks, strategies, and ideas to beat my arthritis or manage pain in non-traditional ways.
- I could become more tolerant to my pain and less dependent on drugs (I can joke about it now . . . pain was my friend while I was arthritic, and I now have a higher tolerance to pain than most people).

- I could extend the time before my body became dependant on the pain meds, and before I needed to move up to stronger meds with greater potential side effects. That would give me more time to find options/solutions before I was forced to take stronger meds, with additional meds to deal with whatever side effects came from them.

I only had to endure three years of pain and pain meds, and I had just started migrating into the much stronger options by the time I beat my arthritis. I consider the timing of my coming out the other side of arthritis very fortunate because I had just months before been prescribed stronger pain relief drugs, due to reaching the maximum daily doses of my previous meds. Those stronger meds resulted in me breaking out in little blisters everywhere on my body, so I had to go back to my earlier meds and tolerate living with a bit more pain because I couldn't increase the dosage anymore.

Ultimately, the pain meds were a tool that I could use when I needed to help me function better. The better I could function, the more I could enjoy the life I did have (which is good for one's soul), and the more energy I could have to fight my arthritis (to find options and try them).

I'm no fan of Western medicine but I accept that it offers another option, and living with less pain is better than living with more pain. I just didn't want to become 100% dependant on the meds . . . and I wanted to delay complications from them for as long as possible. This meant I only ever saw the pain meds as a tool rather than a solution.

It's important to note that if you want to try doing this too, you should make sure you're aware of all of the consequences for you of being off your meds – check with your doctor if you're not sure, particularly if you're further up the pain-management meds list.

Chiropractors, osteopaths, physios, and massage therapists

Sometimes, you might need professional help beyond that offered by doctors or medical practitioners to keep your body moving.

There are some joints you'll struggle to move yourself, or times when you're not sure how to make a joint move without risking hurting yourself even more (particularly your neck: get that wrong and you could end up in a wheelchair – not good). And this is where getting some professional help makes all the difference.

I sought out a range of manual and physical therapy professionals to help me when my 'use it or lose it' exercises (see 'Use it or lose it', p. 94) weren't working.

In my case, I used the following professionals for the following reasons:

- Chiropractors – to make sure my bones and joints were aligned properly.
- Osteopaths – to make sure my bones, joints, tendons, and muscles were working properly in relation to each other.
- Physiotherapists – to massage, stretch, and strengthen my muscles, tendons, and joints.
- Massage therapists – to help remove knots and release tension in my muscles.

When my neck was really causing me problems, I started with my chiropractor and as those treatments progressed, I worked down the list and started treatments with my osteopath, then my physiotherapist and then my massage therapist.

Each of them knew of the other professionals who were helping, and in each case, I made sure each professional communicated with the others, sharing what they had done and what they were planning on doing, so no one did anything that mucked up any treatments we were trying. It was extremely important to me (as the patient) that everyone was on the same page and working towards the same goal of greater mobility in whatever joint we were focused on.

I also made sure I asked lots of questions so I could personally learn more about the joints we were treating, as well as how I could maintain movement once we'd freed up the stubborn joints.

And today, even though I no longer have arthritis, I still see a massage therapist every three weeks for 90 minutes for a full body massage. I treat this as two things: a time out to disconnect from the world; and preventative 'medicine' to remove tension/stress in muscles I may or may not be looking after properly in my life.

Surgery versus healing naturally

I recall my specialist giving me the option of surgery to help with joints that were in pain and causing me problems. In my case, this was initially the joints in my lower back.

While I did think long and hard about the decision, in the end I chose to reject surgery as an option entirely – no matter how bad things got.

My reasoning was that life gives us our bodies for a reason and every joint, muscle, fibre, organ, or cell functions in unison with every other joint, muscle, fibre, organ, or cell in our respective bodies. If you do anything to change that, there will be a ripple effect throughout your body.

There is a natural balance to things which means you could solve one problem with surgery, but create two or more problems elsewhere in your body. So I believe that fusing my lower spine might have caused problems with my neck and upper spine, and possibly my hips and legs, over years to come.

I also believe that our bodies can heal themselves of any ailment. The real problem is that we're crap at giving our bodies what they need to be able to do that (Western medicine hasn't worked out yet what our bodies need to heal themselves). I wouldn't be surprised if, in years to come, we work out we've been poisoning our bodies through most of our lives.

So even though I may not have known what to give my body to heal itself of arthritis, I wanted to at least have the chance of finding what my body needed before I let surgeons fuse my spine so it would no longer work as it naturally should anymore . . . and possibly stuff up the chances of my body healing itself in the process.

Just one final thought on surgery. Even though I believe in balance and natural healing, surgery may be necessary in certain cases – everyone is unique. I just viewed surgery as my plan Z if everything else failed.

Your Body

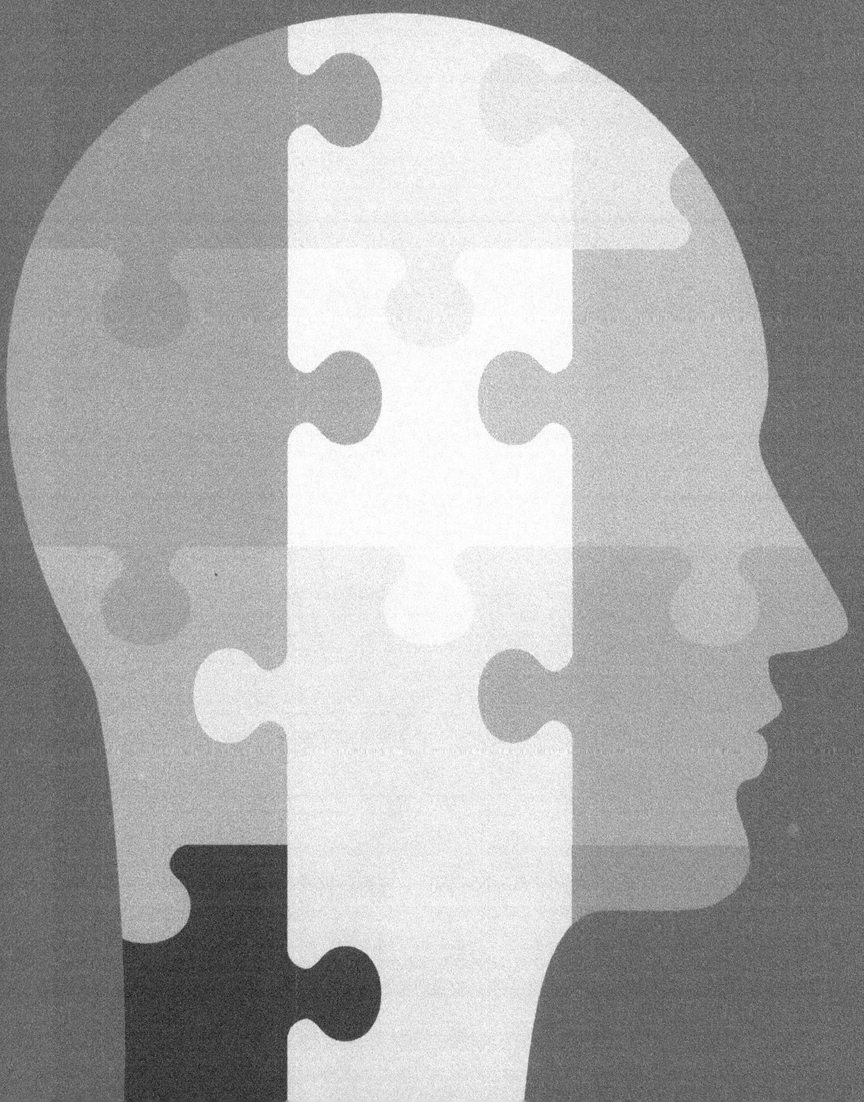

You are what you eat

It seems to me that everyone has a theory about arthritis and food. Friends and family were not shy in sharing their stories about people they knew whose arthritis got worse when they ate tomatoes, or red meat, or something else.

Respecting that each and every person has a unique biology and physiology, it is extremely difficult to really understand what foods may contribute to or reduce inflammation in any specific human body.

However, from the information I read, it seemed clear to me that there must be a link between what we consume and inflammation. I decided that the best way to see how the food I consumed might affect my arthritis was to test the food I ate against the severity of my arthritis at any one time.

Given that my arthritis could fluctuate on an hourly basis, I needed to make sure that whatever foods I consumed could be directly linked to the severity of my arthritis, or lack thereof. The only way I could see to do this was to wean myself off all foods down to basically nothing, and then gradually introduce one food at a time over three-day periods. And that's exactly what I did.

Over a period of three weeks, I gradually weaned myself off all food, down to an unappetising vitamin drink that was neutral as far as foods went and basically just gave me the minimal vitamins and minerals to keep my body going. I remember that it was like drinking wet sawdust.

Having weaned myself off food and living on that unappetising vitamin drink for three days, I then reintroduced one food every three days (my first food was potatoes, and I remember that because I love potatoes). As I introduced each food, I paid close attention to my body and the level of arthritis that I was having to endure.

The moment I got bloated, started farting or burping, or my pain spiked, I would remove that current food for three more days to see what happened. It is important to note I didn't do anything unusual during this period (e.g., no physical exercise other than normal everyday walking). I needed to make sure any bodily reactions were food-related and nothing else.

It's also important to note that when I reintroduced a food, I introduced that food and nothing else. For example, when I started eating potatoes again, they were plain boiled potatoes – no butter, no salt, no spices, no oil. If you react to one food, you need to be 100% sure it's that food only causing the reaction, and not a garnish or flavour enhancer.

Only after three days of enjoying plain potatoes with no ill effects could I look at crispy oven-baked potatoes with some oil, or sliced/diced potatoes pan-fried in oil. And it was another three days before I could introduce salt, and another three days before I could introduce anything else. You get the picture.

The conclusion of my research on myself was that gluten made me worse. My pain was sharper and more intense while eaten gluten. When I removed gluten from my diet, the pain that I had to endure softened and reduced.

It was a pretty easy decision for me. No more gluten.

Even though removing gluten from my diet was a no brainer due to the change in the pain I experienced, I wanted to understand more about why gluten might be bad for me.

In my case, most of the gluten I used to consume was from flour – bread and pasta were a big part of my pre-arthritis diet. So I dug around online, looking for any information about problems with diets, autoimmune problems and inflammation related to flour and gluten. Through this, I uncovered some interesting observations relevant to flour:

- Contemporary milling processes – used since about 1900 – remove the nutritionally important fibre and many natural vitamins and nutrients of the wheat. These are then replaced by vitamins and minerals manufactured in chemical plants.

- Too much change in too short a time frame – the evolution of flour since 1900, and the removal of the 'bits' that were considered unattractive to the final flour product has resulted in a final product that is much finer (smaller) than it was prior to 1900.

- Genetic modification of the plant – today's wheat plant has been modified to resist disease and bugs, and improve yields.

The end result is the wheat plants our grandparents once enjoyed were very different to the wheat we now enjoy in the 21st century.

And while I have no evidence to back this up, I believe that these factors – the replacement of natural vitamins and minerals removed in milling with manufactured ones, the magnitude of change to refined flour in such a short time, modifications made to wheat to resist disease and bugs, along with the increased consumption of flour in Western diets – are each and all likely to have some effect on our digestive system (and on our overall physical wellbeing).

Whether it's the possibility of such finely refined flour escaping the digestive system through leaky gut, potential toxins that protect wheat from bugs and disease even partially surviving the refinement and baking processes, or the introduction of manufactured vitamins and minerals to replace natural ones lost in milling . . . this has happened in such a short period of time that our digestive systems have not had enough time to adapt to so much change to a 'food' that makes up such a large portion of many people's diets.

Whether what I believe about flour and our digestive systems is right or not, I prefer to be safer rather than sorry. So even though I am arthritis-free today, I am happy to remain gluten-free (and white flour-free) to lessen the risks and stress (perceived or otherwise) on my digestive system due to the above.

There is also quite a lot of research and information that points the finger at starch contributing to inflammation.[5]

---

5 One book I found useful regarding this was *The IBS Low-Starch Diet: Why Starchy Food May Be Hazardous to Your Health* by Carol Sinclair (London: Vermillion, 2003).

You might want to try reducing starch in your diet too, if gluten doesn't make a difference for you. There are plenty of books and information online about starch to help you work out how to detect starch in what you eat.

As I mentioned earlier, each human body is unique and – I believe – tuned to prefer and/or dislike specific food groups based on the accessibility of food to your ancestors. So you're going to have to test removing gluten and/or starch from your diet to determine whether that might be a contributing factor to your inflammation and pain. Just because gluten was something that worsened my arthritis, it doesn't necessarily mean that gluten is contributing to your inflammation. That's the beauty and the curse of being human – we're all unique.

The other thing I'd suggest is looking at any foods that have numbers in the ingredients (i.e., processed foods) and processed sugars. There has been lots of research done about how these things impact our bodies – the good and the bad. For me, simply going back to basics and eating natural foods (thereby removing anything artificial which the human body may not deal with so well) seemed logical.

It's also important to note that if you decide to make any significant changes to your diet, including an elimination diet like I tried, please ensure you get medical advice. I was able to do my detox and testing without medical help, but in hindsight that wasn't very smart. Lots of things could have gone wrong by removing so much food from my diet over an extended period. You may have issues removing foods (and the vitamins, proteins, minerals, etc., contained within) down to the point I did; issues that could make your arthritis worse.

Use it or lose it

I don't remember where I originally picked up the phrase 'use it or lose it', but I know it has stuck with me for a long time.

When I became arthritic, the research I did highlighted that while there are different types of arthritis, one thing was common: the sufferer was in pain and movement hurt. If the painful joint was 'protected' by not moving it, that joint would stop working properly due to its reduced range of motion, and ultimately would 'fuse' and no longer work at all.

If I was going to beat my arthritis, I wanted as much range of motion as possible in all my joints.

I believe there are drugs and supplements you can take that are supposed to help with joint mobility. I never took them so I can't share any experience in that area, but you might want to look into this to help prolong your joint mobility while trying to heal yourself. Just don't forget to talk with your health professional first, just in case any supplements impact whatever medication you might be taking.

What I did do, though, was make another conscious choice to protect the range of motion of all joints in my body as much as possible . . . and I accepted the consequences of that choice: moving joints that may be affected by arthritis would be painful.

Instead of doing all the physical exercise I used to do, I sought out alternative range of motion exercises that didn't result in big pain spikes or inflammation in my body. For me, that meant yoga. Tai chi was another one if I wanted to do something different. There are many other options if either of these don't work for you – just check online.

I also used health professionals to help assist any joints under attack from my arthritis, to maintain or improve their range of motion (see 'Chiropractors, osteopaths, physios, and massage therapists', p. 80).

By accepting some pain while keeping my joints moving, I was able to reduce the chances of any part of my body not working as it should when/If I beat my arthritis.

In my case, after three years of living with arthritis and coming out the other side arthritis-free, I can tell you I've only got two parts of my body that don't function as they did before arthritis: one is minor, one knuckle on the end of my little finger on my left hand (it's a bit knobbly, like a witch's finger), and the other is my manubriosternal joint (the bone your ribs attach to at the front of your chest).

Nowadays I have to be careful doing any chest exercises, and balancing those out with back exercises to avoid pressure on the front of my chest . . . but that's a lot better than it could have been, considering I had periods when I was arthritic where my neck was very unhappy and didn't want to turn at all, and my knees and ankles struggled to function.

I know, with 100% certainty, if I hadn't worked as hard on maintaining movement (despite the discomfort that came with joints that didn't want to move), my knees, ankles and neck would be causing me major problems today, even after my arthritis left me.

So regardless of your situation, I believe you must keep moving your joints – both the good ones not suffering inflammation, as well as those joints that could be inflamed. Just do it respectfully to your body and joints – softly and slowly! And even if your journey takes longer than my three years, you'll enjoy greater freedom than if you stop moving your joints and let them seize up.

Use it or lose it – the choice is yours.

Genetics and environmental factors

Prior to 2003, I didn't have arthritis. For whatever reason, from 2003 I did. Any number of things may have contributed to my arthritis activating. Those contributing factors could have been external (what I ate and how I used my body), and/or internal (dumb luck and the genetics I inherited from my parents).

While searching online for more information about arthritis, and ankylosing spondylitis specifically, I found occasional references to a protein called HLA-B27 and its link to arthritis.

Basically, the link went like this:

- HLAs (or human leukocyte antigens) are proteins found on white blood cells in all humans.

- HLAs help our immune system to distinguish between healthy body tissue – cells that belong in the body – and foreign tissue or cells which may lead to disease.

- HLA-B27 is a specific type of HLA protein that has links with immune system problems.

- Not everyone has the gene which causes the specific HLA-B27 protein to develop – it's estimated that approximately 8% of the general population have it.

- The HLA-B27 protein on white blood cells can confuse the immune system and cause it to attack otherwise normal, healthy cells.

- When your body attacks normal, healthy cells, this can result in autoimmune diseases such as ankylosing spondylitis.

What I found most interesting was that not everyone who has the gene which causes the HLA-B27 protein to develop, or who has the HLA-B27 protein present in their blood, has autoimmune problems. Less than 5% of HLA-B27-positive people ever develop ankylosing spondylitis.

This means that just being genetically predisposed to producing the HLA-B27 protein isn't enough to result in you developing arthritis. Something needs to trigger the gene to cause an autoimmune response.

So I won the genetic lottery! I inherited the HLA-B27 gene from one or both of my parents (of the 8% of people in the world carrying that gene) AND sometime leading up to 2003, my immune system somehow got confused and started attacking healthy cells (meaning I was one of the less than 5% of HLA-B27-positive people who develop ankylosing spondylitis).

Lucky me!

Research[6] into how HLA-B27 is triggered indicates that certain bacterial infections could lead to this autoimmune response, specifically:

---

6 Padmini Parameswaran and Michael Lucke, 'HLA B27 Syndromes,' *NCBI Bookshelf* (Treasure Island, FL: StatPearls Publishing, 2021), https://www.ncbi.nlm.nih.gov/books/NBK526043; bpac^{nz}, 'Diagnosis and Management of Axial Spondyloarthritis in Primary Care,' *Best Practice Journal* 76 (2016), https://bpac.org.nz/BPJ/2016/July/spondyloarthritis.aspx; Nicholas J. Sheehan, 'The Ramifications of HLA-B27,' *Journal of the Royal Society of Medicine* 97, no. 1 (January 2004): 10–14, https://doi.org/10.1258/jrsm.97.1.10; John D. Carter, 'Reactive Arthritis,' National Organization for Rare Disorders, https://rarediseases.org/rare-diseases/reactive-arthritis; Eric Gracey and Robert D. Inman, 'Chlamydia-induced ReA: Immune Imbalances and Persistent Pathogens,' *Nature Reviews Rheumatology* 8 (2012): 55–59, https://doi.org/10.1038/nrrheum.2011.173.

- Chlamydia – a sexually transmitted infection caused by bacteria (this didn't apply to me based on my relationship history).

- Salmonella – a common bacteria which lives in the intestinal tract of humans and animals. Infection is most often contracted by eating foods or drinking water contaminated with faeces from an infected animal/person.

- Shigella – a type of bacteria found in human faeces. Infection is spread by touching surfaces contaminated with the bacteria then touching your mouth, or eating contaminated food.

- Yersinia – an infection caused most often by eating raw or undercooked pork contaminated with the Yersinia bacteria.

- Campylobacter – a type of food poisoning that is mainly spread to humans by eating undercooked contaminated meat.

I know in my case I had three severe cases of food poisoning (all from chicken) within a year of me developing my initial symptoms of arthritis. That in itself isn't definitive, and in many ways that's not hugely important because whatever the cause – as I found out later while getting my diagnosis – I was predisposed to autoimmune disorders because I had the HLA-B27 gene . . . and regardless of what happened, I developed the autoimmune disease symptoms sometime in mid-2003.

What is important, though, is not everyone with the HLA-B27 gene develops the haywire autoimmune response leading to arthritic inflammations. There needs to be an environmental trigger to set off the reaction in your body. And this confirmed my initial thoughts that if it can be turned on, then it's logical it could also be turned off . . . if you can find the switch.

Leaky gut

Some of my research around arthritis and autoimmune problems pointed to a condition called 'leaky gut'. If the lining of the small intestine becomes damaged, it can cause undigested food particles, toxic waste products and bacteria to 'leak' through the intestines and flood the bloodstream. This can lead to widespread inflammation and possibly trigger a reaction from the immune system.

Interestingly, some studies[7] have suggested an association

7 Bilal Ahmad Paray, Mohammed Fahad Albeshr, Arif Tasleem Jan, and Irfan A. Rather, 'Leaky Gut and Autoimmunity: An Intricate Balance in Individuals Health and the Diseased State,' *International Journal of Molecular Sciences* 21, no. 24 (2020): 9770, https://doi.org/10.3390/ijms21249770; Veena Taneja, 'Arthritis Susceptibility and the Gut Microbiome,' *FEBS Letters* 588, no. 22 (November 2014): 4244–4249, https://doi.org/10.1016/j.febslet.2014.05.034; Melvin Mashner, 'Can a Leaky Gut Lead to an Autoimmune Condition,' The Gut Authority, https://thegutauthority.com/leaky-gut-and-autoimmune-condition; 'Your Gut's Feeling for Rheumatoid Arthritis – The Leaky Gut Syndrome,' My RA Diary, https://www.myradiary.com/632/your-guts-feeling-for-rheumatoid-arthritis-the-leaky-gut-syndrome.

between leaky gut and autoimmune diseases including arthritis. Unfortunately, there was no conclusive proof as to whether leaky gut contributed to autoimmune problems or whether autoimmune problems contributed to leaky gut.

Despite there being inconclusive research on this topic, I took the approach of improving my diet to include healthier, more natural and less processed foods to help improve my gut lining, bring more balance to my digestive system, and reduce the toxicity of any particles that did leak into my body.

Klebsiella

While researching food and the gut, I fell across another possibility – a specific bacteria called Klebsiella. Klebsiella is a common type of bacteria found in the intestines and faeces of humans, and is generally harmless unless it multiplies too much, or spreads to other parts of the body where it can cause serious infections.

My research[8] indicated:

---

8 Li Zhang et al., 'The Association of HLA-B27 and Klebsiella Pneumoniae in Ankylosing Spondylitis: A Systematic Review,' *Microbial Pathogenesis* 117 (April 2018): 49–54, https://doi.org/10.1016/j.micpath.2018.02.020; Aland Ebringer, 'The Relationship Between Klebsiella Infection and Ankylosing Spondylitis,' *Baillière's Clinical Rheumatology* 3, no. 2 (August 1989): 321–338, https://doi.org/10.1016/S0950-3579(89)80024-X; Todd Mansfield, 'Klebsiella: Ankylosing Spondylitis, Reactive Arthritis & Infections,' Byron Herbalist, https://www.byronherbalist.com.au/gut-health/klebsiella-ankylosing-spondylitis-reactive-arthritis-infections; Chris Kesser, 'HLA-B27 and Autoimmune Disease: Is a Low-Starch Diet the Solution?', https://chriskresser.com/hla-b27-and-autoimmune-disease-is-a-low-starch-diet-the-solution.

- Klebsiella bacteria multiply and flourish when certain foods that typically lead to inflammation, particularly starch and refined carbohydrates, are consumed.

- An overgrowth of the bacteria results in the bacteria, and the toxins the bacteria expel, being more likely to leak from the digestive system into other parts of the body, leading to an inflammatory response.

- Klebsiella bacteria tends to show up in greater numbers in the digestive system of people who had active arthritis.

Much like leaky gut, studies haven't found a conclusive answer whether the bacteria contributes to arthritis, or the arthritis contributes to the incidence of the bacteria. Regardless of what may be true, if the arthritis I was suffering was caused in any way by the presence or overabundance of the bacteria, then it made sense to me to at least try to reduce or remove it from my digestive system. So, I made the decision to starve any Klebsiella that I might have in my digestive tract of the nutrients it liked, and reduced/removed any starch and refined carbohydrate-based foods from my diet.

Purging your body

I recall reading something online about a monastery where foreigners could go to heal, and one of the things visitors had to do was drink some brew they were given that would result in them purging their body at both ends. Apparently, this was to cleanse their system of whatever toxins the modern world had inflicted on them.

While I can't remember all the details now (and unfortunately, I couldn't find this information online again), what is important is a link between this story and the final moments leading up to me being free of arthritis.

In July 2006, I ate the same lunch I had eaten regularly for years – a roast beef or pork meal from a food bar just down the road from where I was working in Auckland. I got food poisoning this time and I ended up spending that night and the next day on the toilet purging from both ends of my body. Not pleasant!

However, what I didn't know at the time was these were my final arthritic moments, because once the purging finished, I was pain-free (and as I would find out later, I was arthritis-free).

It took me about three weeks to realise what had happened because I was just waiting for my pain to come back . . . and it didn't.

Initially, I was very reluctant to take my pain meds after my physical purging because I knew that my stomach and digestive system ideally should take time to heal properly before I subjected them to the possible side effects of the pain meds (particularly the risk of stomach ulcers). So, I delayed taking my pain meds that next day. No pain arrived. I delayed it another day to give my stomach and digestive system more time to heal.

Still no pain.

This continued for about five days before I thought I felt a little niggle coming back and I took my pain meds (I was scared I might end up with a large pain spike for the days I hadn't been in pain AND I needed to take the pills early to bridge the time lag they usually took to kick in).

Because it had been five days before I took that first pill (and that was very unusual because in the past I'd be lucky to function without the pain meds for more than a couple of days), I decided to try not taking the next pill and test whether I was actually in pain anymore.

Three weeks after that first post-purge 'fear' pill, I realised my arthritis was gone, and I stopped looking for the signs of pain returning and instead revelled in being pain-free again.

Sometimes the end is just the beginning

In the years following me becoming arthritis-free, I struggled getting back to exercising regularly like I did before my arthritis.

A large part of that struggle was because I wondered, 'Why bother?' I had lived what I considered an above-average healthy life pre-arthritis and yet at 35 years it still hit me.

In my head, I rationalised my hesitance by asking myself the loaded question: 'What's the point of trying to live healthily if I end up getting arthritic anyway?'

The answer was . . . there was no point. I realised that I may as well just enjoy life and not worry too much about living healthily seeing as it's really just a crap shoot as to what life may throw at you.

Despite thinking such things, I still knew that it was important to exercise regularly, especially to maintain my range of motion and function in my joints and muscles, so I tried to reintroduce exercise into my life. Unfortunately, every time I started to exercise again post-arthritis, I invariably got another injury. And I'd be forced to rest that injury to avoid further problems.

And this then piled back on the question – 'What's the point?' I tried to start exercising . . . and I tried to be careful . . . but I'd get injured . . . and I'd need to stop exercising to treat the injury properly. Head, meet brick wall!

It's taken me many years to get through this and to change my internal dialogue from 'What's the point?' to 'Things have changed – you need to change, too.'

With enough time, and on reflection, the truth behind my injuries was less about life telling me to not bother exercising, and more that:

- I am older and a parent, which slowly wears everything down, so I can't always do today what I used to do pre-arthritis.

- While I was arthritic, my joints and muscles weren't being subjected to resistance, so they weren't required to be as strong nor as flexible as they once were, which means my muscles and joints are no longer used to loading nor resistance.

- The arthritis itself would have affected the joints around my body . . . so that means my joints may not work like they used to. They may not have full range of movement. They may not be able to be loaded under resistance.

The end result was I had to start from scratch again, lifting embarrassingly light weights and using low-resistance exercise bands pre-teenage boys might laugh at. And I had to take things very slowly with the full range of movement for all joints.

I know, physically, I will never have what I used to have pre-arthritis when it comes my fitness or strength. I'm okay with that now. But it has taken a while . . . longer than the three years it took me to beat my arthritis.

Besides, who knows? With any luck, and consistently doing the small things right over a long enough period . . . I could end up physically better than I was pre-arthritis.

I do think it's ironic though – I thought I had beaten my arthritis when my pain was gone after three years. However, the truth is that it's one thing getting through the physical experience of arthritis. It's entirely another dealing with the fallout of having (and for those who make it through, having had) arthritis. Never underestimate the fallout you end up accepting having lived with arthritis . . . and the time/effort needed to deal with that in your head.

Be open to the possibilities

One final thought reflecting on my journey – don't limit yourself.

There's more to life than anyone will ever know. I admit there are things I see and hear that initially seem weird to me and make no sense (which I'd normally dismiss in a heartbeat). However, on further reflection, sometimes the illogical can be logical. For example, I know in a land of the unexpected, you can expect the unexpected. I know something can be perfect due to its imperfections.

Reflecting on my final 'purge', I wondered whether I would have voluntarily induced a purge to 'cure' myself and I still can't answer that question today. While I didn't like dealing with random levels of pain at any time, I'm not a big fan of voluntarily throwing up and getting the shits either. And I must be clear here – I cannot say with certainty that enduring the food poisoning I experienced in July 2006 cured me. My purge was just the final moment when I was released from the grip arthritis had over me.

There is a possibility that I had passed whatever tests life required of me and the purge I endured was not food poisoning at all, but merely a necessary evil before I took my next step in life.

There is also the possibility that to progress to the next level in life, I had to leave the 'old' me behind and be 'reborn' . . . and the purge I went through was that rite of passage.

And there is also the possibility that throwing up and shitting purged my body, removing any/all Klebsiella from my digestive system and thereby removed the cause of toxins leeching into my body.

These are all 'out there' possibilities with little or no scientific basis . . . but I accept there is more to life than any of us will ever understand. And while I am a very logic-based person, I cannot dismiss outright anything that may be 'out there' just because it doesn't fit with what I think I know currently.

There are things we don't know . . . and they might be just as valid (or more valid) than what we think we know. And when you are having to live with pain 24/7 and you don't want to live in pain anymore, anything is worth a shot.

So, what's the secret to beating arthritis?

Now we get to the point of how best to beat your arthritis.

In many ways this may be the most important section in this book, and I suspect some of you have skipped straight to this section, eager to find the conclusion – the cure – to being pain-free and rid of your arthritis.

But, as is the case for me and everything I see in life (being the contrarian I am), this is also the least important section in my book.

Unfortunately, life doesn't offer us an easy off-the-shelf answer.

And if it did, I'd be suspicious.

Using Arthritis Against Itself

Nothing that's worthwhile is easy, and silver bullets tend to be fictions created by snake oil merchants looking to make a quick buck. Humans will always fall for them because everyone wants the most efficient way to get what they want.

I don't want to disappoint you . . . arthritis is no different. There are quacks galore and snake oil merchants selling all sorts of potions and remedies to cure your arthritis and pain. I don't believe in them (in fact, I didn't believe them while forging my own path), and I'm not one of them.

What I bring is experience. I lived with arthritis for three years: in constant pain, starting from a point where trained doctors and quacks alike gave me no hope of being pain-free ever, searching and reviewing volumes of information looking for answers, testing those answers that I believed made some sense on myself, and eventually coming out the other side.

So I believe that makes me more than qualified to talk about what works and what doesn't.

And reflecting on my journey, here is what I think is the ultimate secret to beating arthritis; the one simple rule that will see you come out the other side of your arthritis and be pain-free.

Here goes . . .

There isn't one!

Yes, that's right. If you were looking for a quick fix then I'm sorry to disappoint you. There is no big secret except for maybe this . . .

> *'If something is possible for any other man, it is possible for you too.'*
> *—Marcus Aurelius*

I never knew I could get rid of my arthritis, either temporarily or permanently. Yet here I am today – arthritis-free since mid-2006!

Regardless of how long you have had arthritis, regardless of the level of pain meds you are now on, and regardless of what anyone may have told you, you're already one step closer to being arthritis-free than I was when I started – you know I did it. I beat my arthritis. And that means it's possible you can do it too.

And you can get another step closer by learning from my insights. Read the rest of my book (if you haven't already) to become aware of what, why and how I did what I did to come out the other side and beat my arthritis. Everything I shared is replicable by you, as long as you have the desire and persistence to apply them in your life.

I believe unlocking your secret to coming out the other side of arthritis is more like a combination lock than a padlock. You're going to have to find the right combination of life choices to turn it off and/or starve it to death . . . as opposed to finding the *one* thing that will work.

Anything more to add?

There hasn't been a day since July 2006 that I haven't been grateful for having beaten my arthritis.

And at the same time, there hasn't been a day since then that I haven't asked myself the following two questions:

- If I could change my past, would I change it so I never had arthritis at all?

- What would I have done if I hadn't beaten my arthritis when I did?

Let me start by saying I wouldn't change my past to have never had arthritis. Yes, it sucked. But it is only because of arthritis that I know with 100% certainty that anything is possible despite what anyone tells you. You just have to want it enough to do whatever is necessary to make it happen.

I also appreciate what it feels like to live with pain 24/7, so I have a lot more respect and empathy for others who endure arthritis or other autoimmune problems.

Now when I see someone limping down the road towards me, I ALWAYS make way for them because I know it's easier for me to change direction than it may be for them. And I never try and help someone without asking them if they would like my help first.

If I hadn't beaten my arthritis, I know with 100% certainty I wouldn't have stopped, and I'd still be trying other strategies today to reduce my pain. I would have kept researching medical journals to keep up to date with research as new links were found. I'd be testing that research on myself (with medical support if relevant). And I'd probably be digging around ideas that are more spiritual and less conscious, looking for old wisdom from more 'fringe' healers. Giving up isn't in my bones.

So if you (the reader) have arthritis and/or you are living in pain 24/7, I want you to know that I know your pain – both the pain you endure in your body as well as all the noise that comes with that in your head.

Whether you have medical support that gives you hope or not, I truly believe a pain-free life can be yours too, if you can find your path. I acknowledge what I have shared with you was my path. I know, unfortunately, that it may not work for you. However, what I do know is all these experiences I've shared with you contributed to my result, and they will at the very least give you ideas to help reduce your pain and reliance on modern medicine. And at best, they may help you find your path through whatever autoimmune disease you are facing.

I wish you all the best with your journey. My hope is one day we understand what is truly going on that causes so many of the autoimmune messes in our bodies, so people don't have to endure pain 24/7 like I had to (and you have to).

Enduring pain 24/7 is a big cross to bear in life over and on top of living in general. No one who lives without pain will ever understand that. You have my respect carrying that burden . . . even more so if you do find your way through this and come out the other side.

And if you do make it to the other side, you should know that life becomes a walk in the park because you no longer have to endure the pain you had to, nor the crap that came with that. You will be able to handle so much more than 'normal' people, having carried that cross of pain.

I wish you all the best on your journey, and if/when you do successfully make it through, I would love to hear from you. You can email me at brydon@infinitepossibilities.co.nz.

Epilogue

After two months of being pain-free, I decided to do one final thing to double-check I was really free. I went back to my specialist to get retested. Those tests came back all clear – not one arthritic marker was positive anymore. I was truly free of arthritis!

I remember my specialist telling me those results from behind his desk . . . and I remember he also told me that my arthritis could come back. I felt like slapping him senseless at the time because at the beginning of my journey he never said it could go away, only that I'd have to live with it for the rest of my life. He never gave me any hope – I had to make my own hope.

I left his office with one very clear thought. Whether my arthritis could or would come back didn't matter to me. I was pain-free that day (and had been for two glorious months) and I was going to make the most of every day . . . as opposed to living in fear it could come back.

Not only that, but if it did come back . . . I've beaten it once already, so I know it's possible to do it again.

www.ingramcontent.com/pod-product-compliance
Lightning Source LLC
Chambersburg PA
CBHW072144020426
42334CB00018B/1885
* 9 7 8 0 4 7 3 6 2 1 0 1 8 *